Home Health Nurse Notes

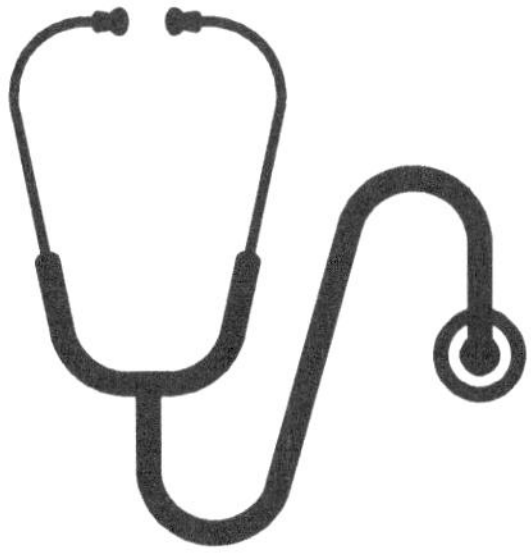

This book belongs to:

____

Coloring Section

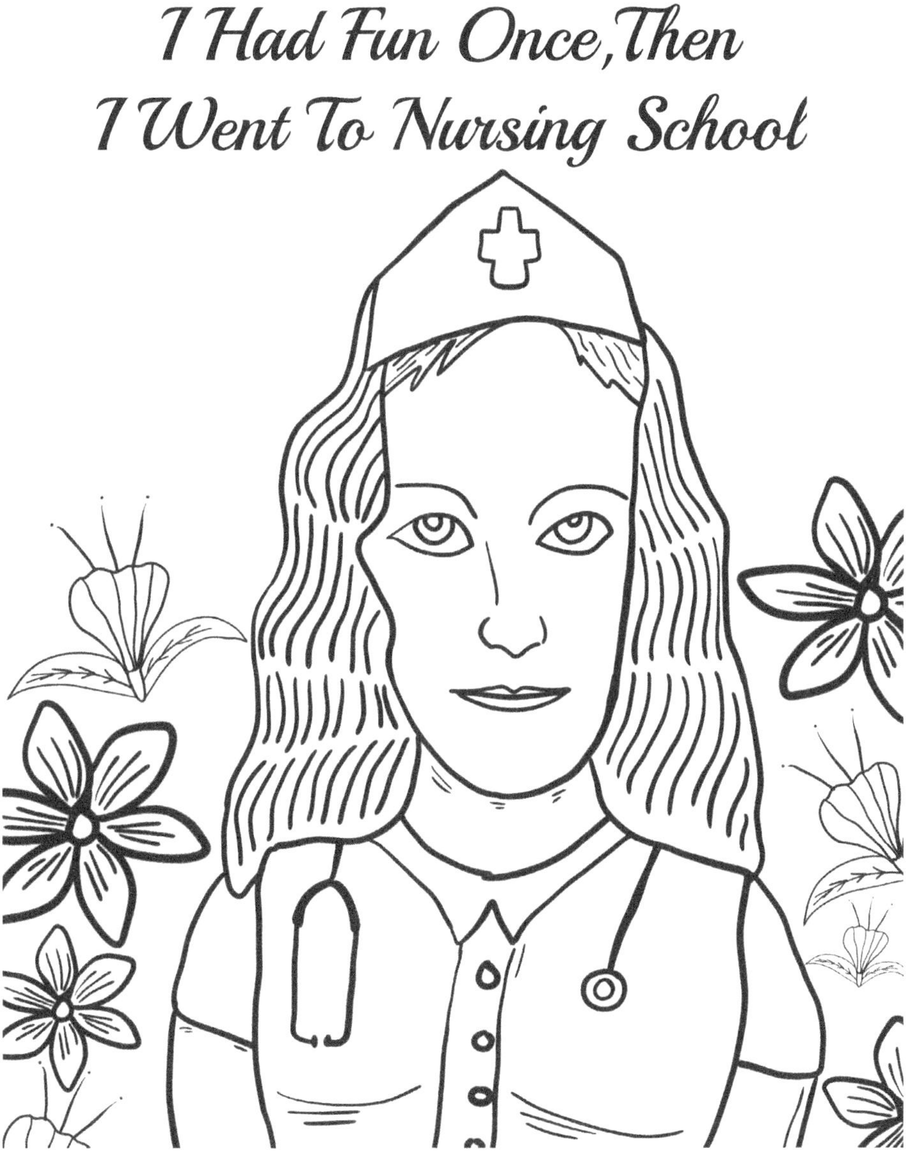

Ativan A Nurse's Best Friend

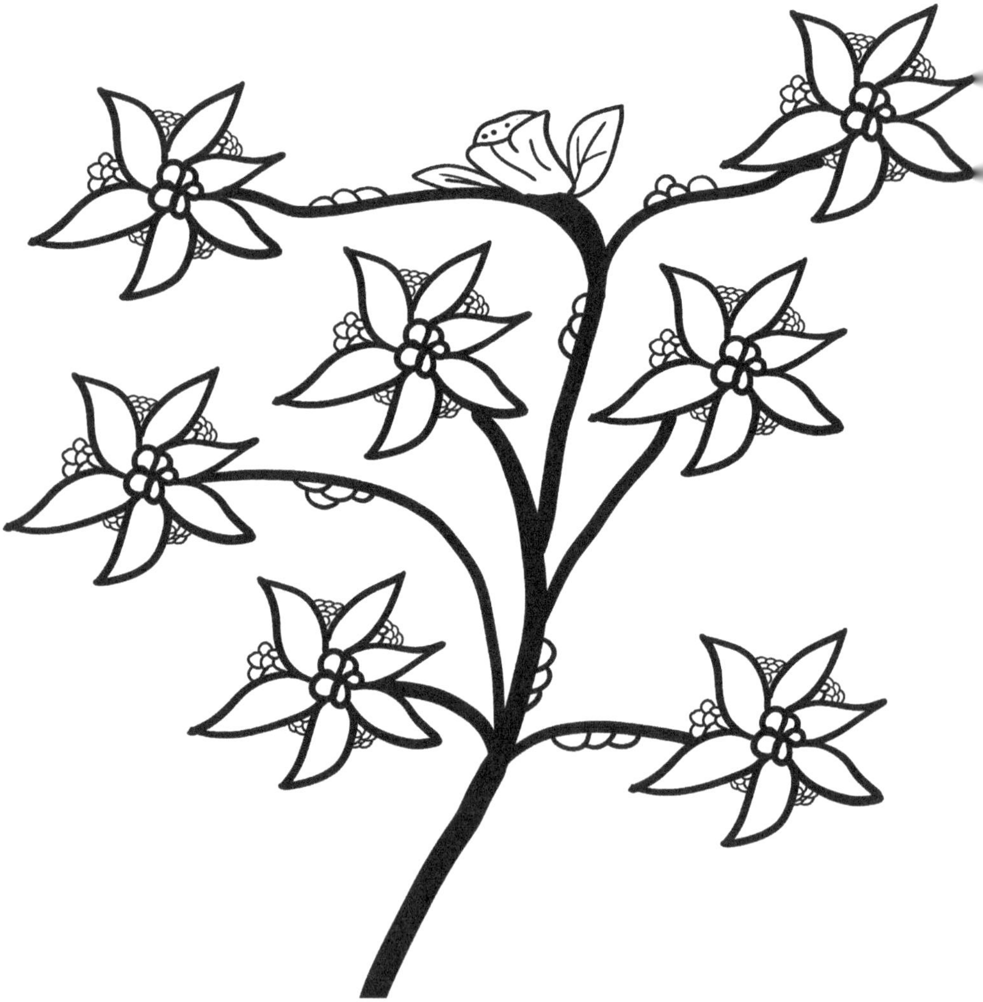

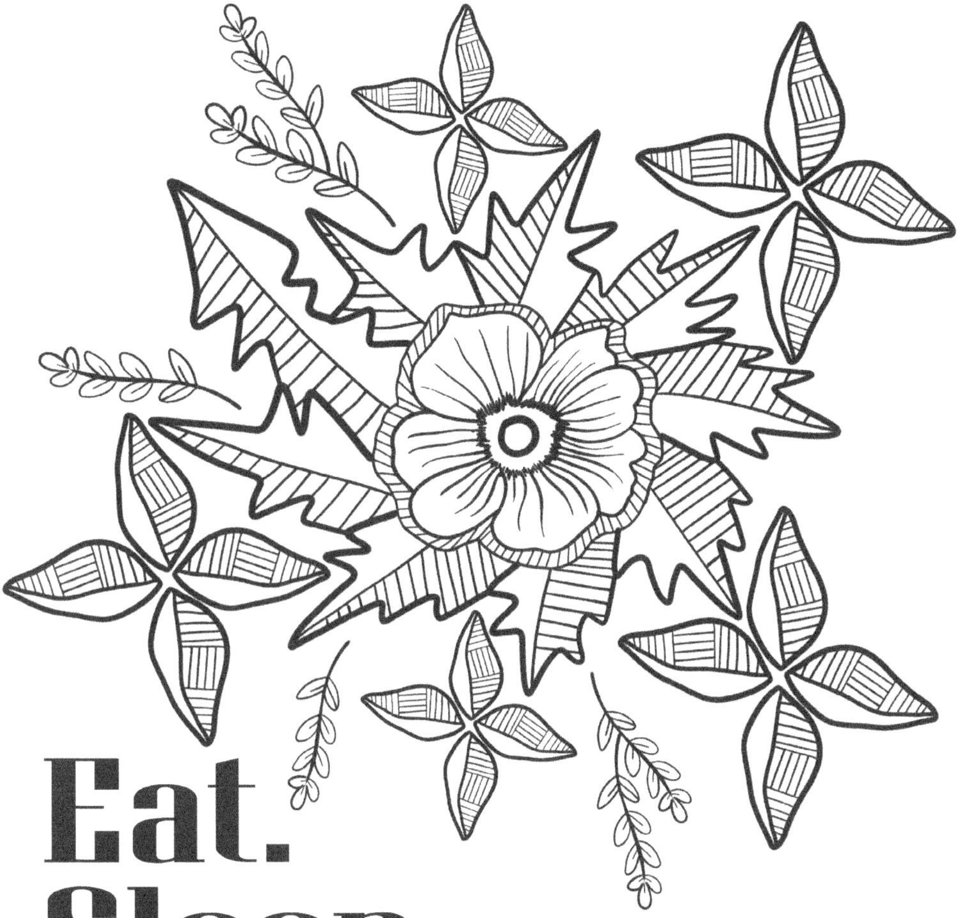

Eat.
Sleep.
Nurse.
Repeat

Do Not Make Me Sedate You.

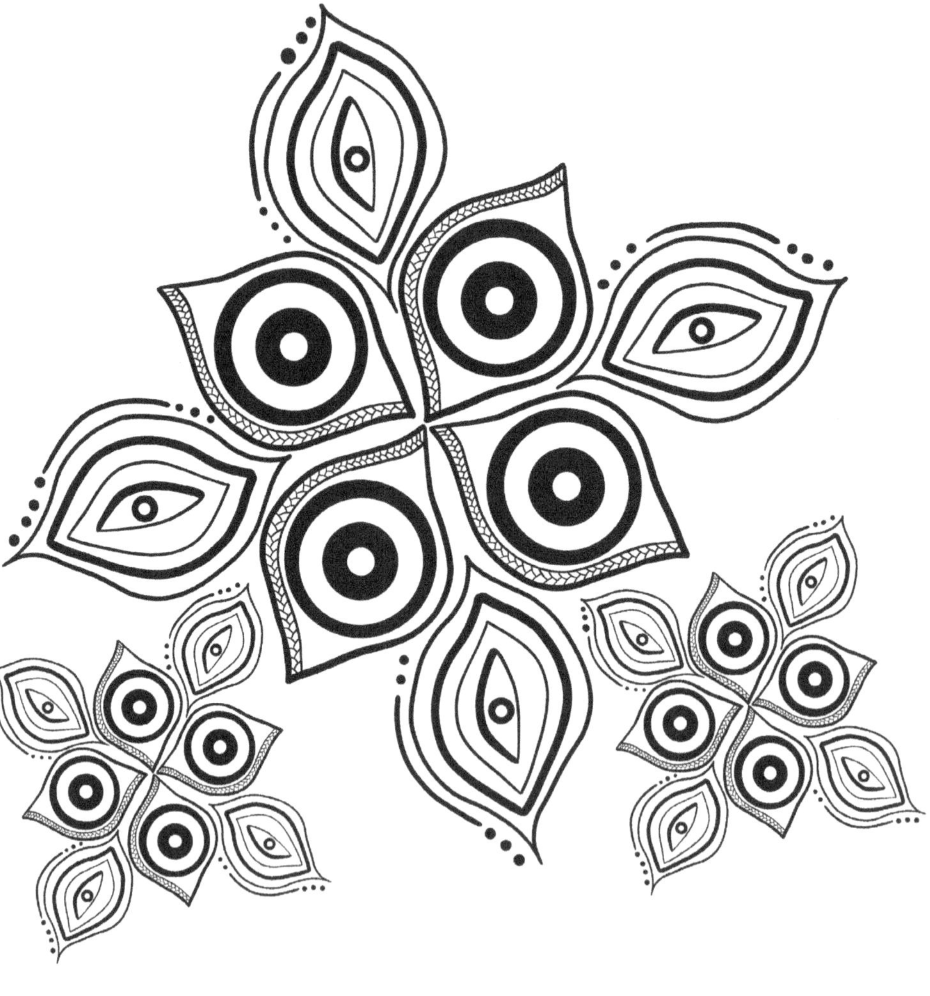

Best Nurse Ever

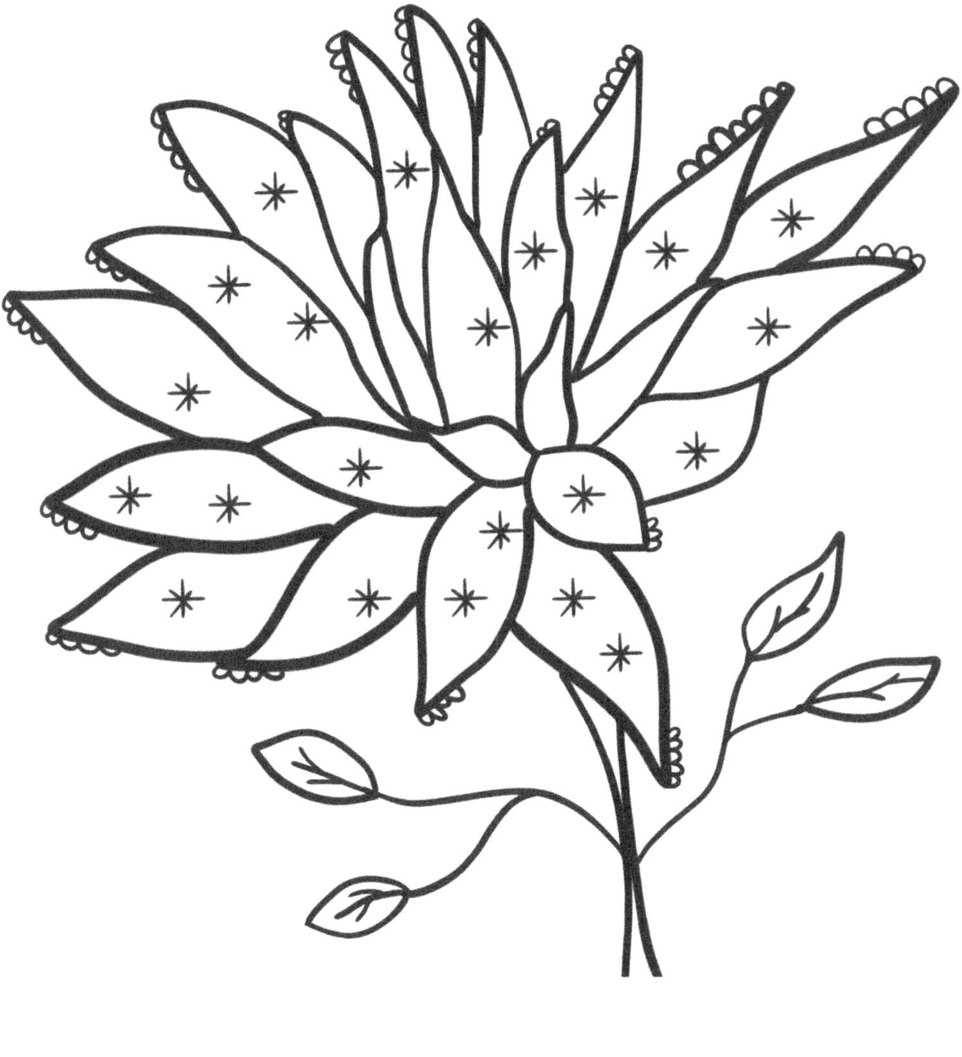

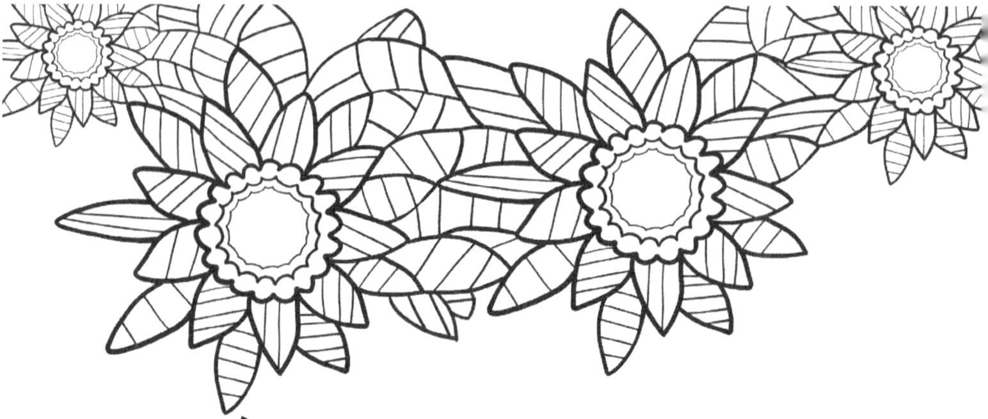

I'VE SEEN MORE PRIVATES THAN THE ARMY GENERAL

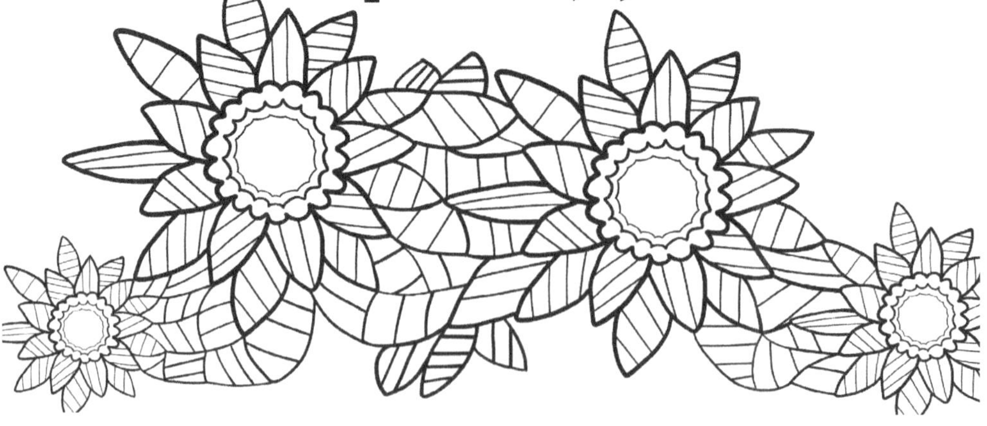

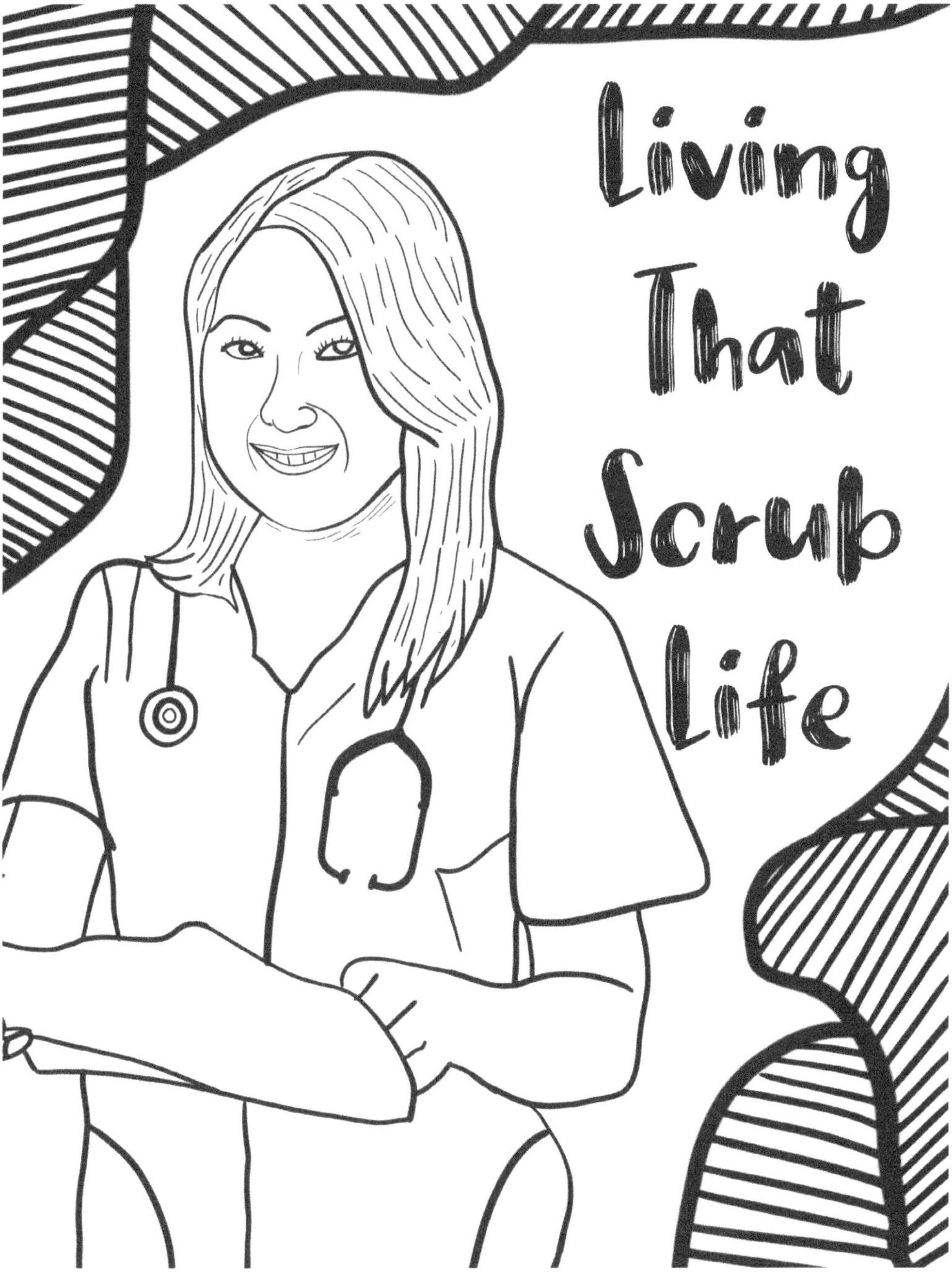
Living
That
Scrub
Life

Nurse Squad

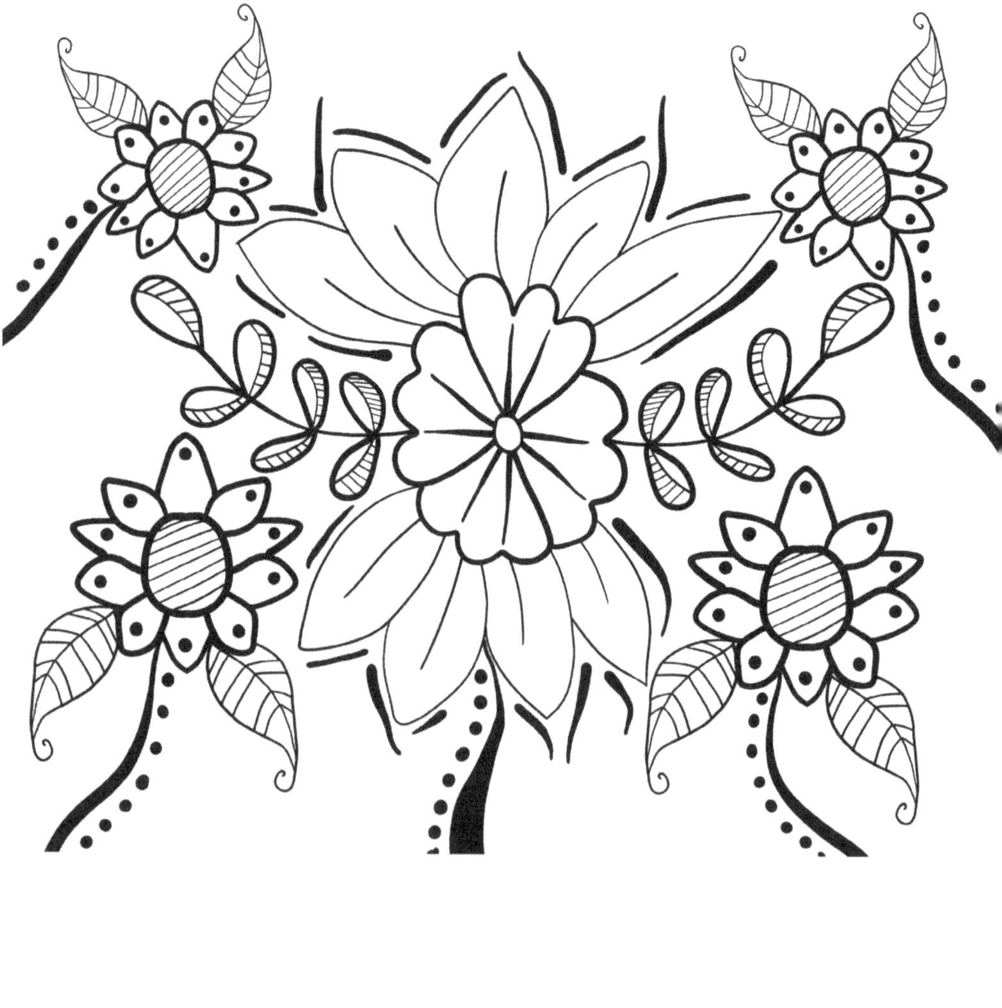

If You're Happy and You Know It, It's Your Meds

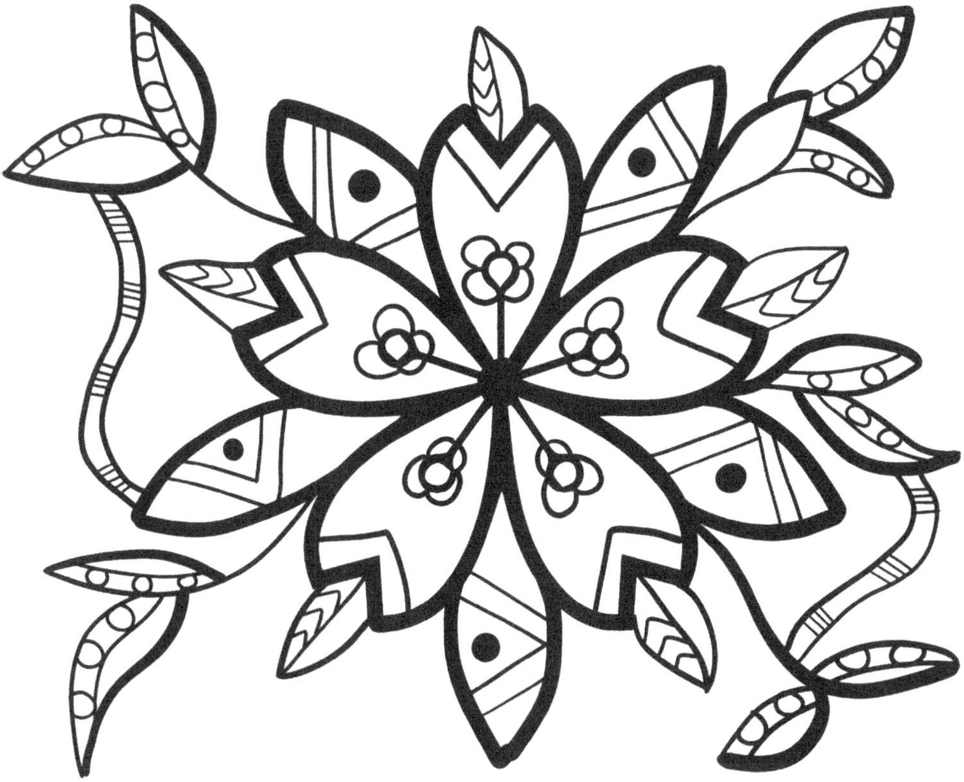

www.ingramcontent.com/pod-product-compliance
Lightning Source LLC
Chambersburg PA
CBHW070438180526
45158CB00019B/1652
9781087417509